I0706938

The Power of Good Energy

A Simple and Effective Method to Enhance Your Well-Being and Happiness

By

Dwight W. Gagne

DISCLAIMER

Copyright © by Dwight W. Gagne 2024. All rights reserved. Before this document is duplicated or reproduced in any manner, the publisher's consent must be gained. Therefore, the contents within can neither be stored electronically, transferred, nor kept in a database. Neither in Part nor full can the document be copied, scanned, faxed, or retained without approval from the publisher or creator.

Table of Contents

Introduction

What Is Good Energy, and why Does It Matter?

Have you ever experienced sudden feelings of exhaustion, worry, or unhappiness? Have you ever questioned why certain people seem to exude charisma, attraction, and a natural glow? Have you ever hoped for a happier, healthier, and more satisfying life?

This book is for you if any of these questions apply to you. In this book, you will learn about the power of positive energy and how it can completely change your life.

What constitutes positive energy? The uplifting, lively, and harmonious force that permeates our surroundings and lives is known as good energy. It is life itself, the source of happiness, and the impetus behind achievement. It serves as our link to the cosmos, to other people, and ourselves.

Why is positive energy important? Positive energy influences everything we do, think, feel, and encounter, which is why it counts. It affects our relationships, creativity, productivity, well-being, and sense of purpose. It determines our fate and shapes our world.

How do we get and make use of positive energy? This book will teach you how to access and utilize positive energy in a variety of ways, including:

How to connect your aspirations and objectives with the strength of your mind, body, and soul.

How to make a positive influence on others as well as oneself by radiating and attracting positive energy.

How to deal with difficulties and misfortune, as well as get over negative energy and stress.

How to preserve the environment and its resources by using renewable energy sources.

This book isn't a miracle cure or an easy fix. It is a friend, a tool, and a guide on your journey of self-improvement. It is founded on empirical studies, common sense, and firsthand accounts. It is intended to uplift, empower, and encourage you to lead a happier, healthier, and more contented life.

Are you prepared to experience good energy's power? So let's get going!

Chapter One

The Science of Energy: How Everything is Connected by Vibrations.

Every part of our lives is impacted by the basic concept of energy, which also shapes the universe in invisible ways. At the center of this complicated dance of forces is the deep idea that everything is related through vibrations. This idea, which has its roots in metaphysics, quantum mechanics, and physics, reveals an intriguing tapestry that ties reality together.

We must explore the domains of physics, where particles and waves are considered to be the fundamental building blocks of matter, to fully understand the science of energy. Particles at the subatomic scale have dual natures, acting as waves and as distinct entities. The idea of vibrations is introduced by this wave-particle duality, in which particles oscillate in rhythmic patterns to produce an energy symphony that goes beyond the limits of the material universe.

The fundamental idea of this networked dance is that energy is vibrational. Every object in the universe vibrates at a different frequency, which results in a harmonic resonance that reverberates over time and space. This global rhythm is the foundation of everything, from the largest cosmic structures to the tiniest subatomic particles.

The idea of energy quantization arises in quantum mechanics, the study of matter's tiniest particles. Energy levels are distinct, and energy quanta are exchanged during transitions between these levels. This quantization highlights the tiny interconnectivity of energy and is closely related to the vibrational modes of particles.

Beyond the domain of quantum mechanics, classical physics presents the idea of waves and their function in explaining the movement of energy. Waves' frequency and amplitude properties make them an effective tool for studying how energy moves across different media. The fundamental idea behind all motion, whether it be the massive waves of the ocean or the soft ripples in a pond, is that energy is transferred through vibrations.

Beyond the boundaries of the material world, into the metaphysical and spiritual realms, energy vibrations are being studied. Energy has long been used by ancient wisdom traditions to realize the interconnection of all things. Eastern philosophies emphasize the flow of life energy through the body, which connects each individual being to the larger universe. Examples of these concepts are

Qi in Chinese medicine and Prana in Indian philosophy.

In the realm of music and sound, vibrations are paramount. All those musical notes are the vibrations of molecules of air, which combine to produce melodies and harmonies that appeal to our emotions. The visual depiction of sound vibrations is further demonstrated by the study of cymatics, which reveals complex patterns created by materials exposed to various frequencies. The significant influence vibrations have on forming the physical universe is highlighted by this visual representation.

The concept of everything being interconnected via vibrations is not exclusive to the microscopic or metaphysical domains; it also encompasses the celestial bodies that make up our world. The universe is a gigantic vibrating symphony, with planets, stars, and galaxies all participating in the cosmic dance. According to Einstein's general theory of relativity, gravitational waves are rippling effects in spacetime brought on by huge objects accelerating. These waves, which have been observed recently, offer concrete proof that the universe is active and vibrating.

Gaining an understanding of vibrational energy research has benefits in many different industries. Ultrasonography is a medical procedure that uses the vibrational characteristics of sound waves to make inside body components visible. Similar to this, MRI and other technologies use atoms' magnetic resonance to produce finely detailed images. These breakthroughs in medicine demonstrate the significant influence of this scientific understanding of vibrational energy on human health.

Quantum entanglement is a new field that expresses the idea of vibrational interconnectivity. No matter how far apart two particles are, their states are coupled when they become entangled. Classical concepts of space and time are subverted when one particle's state changes instantaneously and impacts the other. This event highlights the vibrating threads that bind the universe together, underscoring the profound connectedness that extends beyond physical isolation. Technology-wise, quantum computing uses the concepts of superposition and entanglement to do calculations at a rate that is not possible for traditional computers. Quantum bits, or qubits, which exist in several states simultaneously, take the place of bits in traditional computing. By pushing the limits of computing power, these quantum states can be manipulated thanks to the complex dance of vibrations occurring at the quantum level.

There are connections between environmental consciousness and the study of energy and vibrations. The vibrational energy lens can be used to understand the interdependence of ecosystems, patterns of climate, and the fragile balance of nature. Ecological imbalances and climate change result from human activities that upset this delicate equilibrium by releasing vibrations in the form of pollutants and emissions. Encouraging sustainable coexistence with the world requires an understanding of and commitment to reducing these vibrational repercussions. Vibrations provide the physics of energy to tell a fascinating story of connection. The rhythmic dance of energy shapes the very fabric of existence, from the microscopic world of quantum particles to the gigantic scale of celestial bodies.

This knowledge cuts beyond academic boundaries and has an impact on a wide range of industries, including technology, physics, medicine, and spirituality. Accepting the significant implications of vibrational connection promotes a more comprehensive understanding of the intricate symphony that binds everything in the vast cosmic tapestry and provides a holistic perspective on our existence.

1.The Power of the Mind: How to Cultivate Positive Thoughts and Emotions.

The mind is a potent instrument that can affect our success, pleasure, and general well-being. But a lot of people have bad feelings and ideas that can prevent them from reaching their objectives and leading happy lives. Thankfully, there are strategies for developing a positive outlook that can support us in overcoming obstacles, managing stress, and appreciating the here and now. Putting more emphasis on our positive traits and strengths than on our shortcomings and defects is one of the most important steps toward cultivating a happy mindset. We may increase our self-confidence and self-esteem as well as inspire ourselves to follow our passions and interests by acknowledging and valuing our strengths. Additionally, we may make a positive impact on the world and assist others by using our strengths, which can strengthen our sense of meaning and purpose.

Engaging in acts of gratitude and self-compassion is crucial for developing a happy outlook. Being grateful means not whining about what we don't have but expressing thanks for what we do have. We may strengthen our happy feelings, including joy, love, and fulfillment, by being grateful for the people, things, and experiences that make our lives better. We can also lessen our bad feelings, such as frustration, bitterness, and jealousy. Being kind and understanding to ourselves, especially when we experience hardships or make mistakes, is the act of practicing self-compassion. We may improve our self-acceptance and self-forgiveness and decrease our self-judgment and self-criticism by being compassionate with ourselves.

Finding the bright side and appreciating the present is a third strategy for developing a cheerful outlook. Seeking the good in every circumstance, especially when things seem hopeless or go wrong, is known as "finding the silver lining." By doing this, we can develop from our experiences, learn from our mistakes, and adjust to our current situation. To truly savor the moment, one must be aware of and grateful for the good things that occur in life, such as a stunning sunset, a delectable meal, or a comforting hug. We can improve our happiness, gratitude, and awareness by doing this.

We can harness the enormous power of the mind to our benefit by developing an optimistic outlook. We can increase our well-being, happiness, and success by concentrating on our good traits and strengths, cultivating self-compassion and thankfulness, and looking for the bright side of things while appreciating the present. We may cultivate and sustain a positive mindset with practice and effort; it's not something we're born with. Thus, let's begin now and develop a lifelong habit of optimistic thinking that will help us.

2. The Power of the Body: How to Boost Your Physical Energy and Health.

Sustaining good physical energy and health is essential in the fast-paced world of today, where demands on our time and attention seem limitless. Our total well-being is greatly influenced by the power of our bodies, which affects not only our physical health but also our mental and emotional fortitude. We'll talk about how to improve physical energy and health in this session, covering everything from the value of consistent exercise to the impact of diet and sleep.

Physical Activity: The Basis of Physical Power

Frequent exercise is essential to leading a healthy lifestyle. Exercise has a major impact on our mental health, in addition to strengthening our muscles and cardiovascular system. Our bodies release endorphins, also referred to as "feel-good" hormones, when we exercise. These hormones help us feel happier and less stressed.

Exercise regimens and intensities might differ depending on personal preferences and medical problems. Finding a workout that fits with one's interests, whether it be weightlifting, yoga, brisk walking, or running, enhances the likelihood of long-term commitment. Including physical exercise in regular activities, such as walking during breaks or using the stairs rather than the elevator, can help boost energy levels.

Fueling the Body for Optimal Performance: Nutrition

Our bodies use the food we eat as fuel, which affects how well they can function. To sustain general health and energy levels, a diet rich in nutrients and balance is necessary. Consuming a range of fruits, vegetables, whole grains, lean proteins, and healthy fats gives you the nutrition you need to stay energized all day. Although it's sometimes overlooked, staying hydrated is essential for sustaining energy levels. Fatigue and reduced cognitive performance can result from dehydration. It is essential to maintain a sufficient intake of water, herbal teas, and other hydration drinks to support the body's numerous processes.

Restorative and Rejuvenating Effects of Good Sleep

Enough sleep is occasionally forfeited in the name of living a hectic life. However, getting enough sleep is essential for both mental and physical health. The body goes through important processes, including hormone regulation, memory consolidation, and muscle restoration, when you sleep. Prolonged sleep deprivation weakens the immune system and decreases cognitive function, rendering people more susceptible to sickness.

Better sleep quality is a result of establishing a regular sleep schedule, making your bedroom cozy, and avoiding stimulants like caffeine just before bed. Putting sleep at the top of your list of priorities for general health and realizing its significance can make a big difference in your resilience and physical energy.

Stress Reduction: Keeping the Body and Mind in Balance

Although stress is an inherent aspect of life, prolonged stress can have negative effects on one's physical and emotional well-being. Creating efficient stress-reduction strategies is essential to preserving equilibrium. Deep breathing techniques, mindfulness meditation, and taking up hobbies are a few practices that might reduce stress and enhance well-being.

Emotional resilience is also enhanced by developing strong social ties and asking for help when necessary. It has been demonstrated that human connection improves mental health by lowering feelings of loneliness and offering a network of support during trying times. Frequent Medical Exams: Preventive Maintenance

A proactive approach to preserving physical well-being is known as preventive healthcare. Frequent check-ups facilitate the early identification of possible problems, allowing for prompt management and intervention. Keeping an eye on vital health metrics, like blood pressure, cholesterol, and blood sugar, enables people to make educated lifestyle decisions and handle any new health issues.

Making preventative healthcare a regular part of one's routine shows a dedication to long-term health. It entails working together with medical specialists to create individualized plans for preserving and enhancing health.

Holistic Methods: Combining the Spirit, Body, and Mind

A comprehensive understanding of the relationship between the mind, body, and spirit is necessary for overall well-being. Exercises like tai chi and yoga not only improve physical strength and flexibility but also mental focus and emotional equilibrium. These holistic methods place a strong emphasis on integrating different facets of health to promote harmony and connectivity.

Increasing bodily energy and well-being requires an understanding of and the ability to use the body's capabilities. People can lay the groundwork for long-term well-being by engaging in regular exercise, eating a healthy, balanced diet, getting enough sleep, effectively managing stress, and supporting preventive healthcare. A holistic approach to health, with an emphasis on mind-body integration, guarantees a thorough and long-lasting influence on an individual's general vigor and ability to bounce back from setbacks.

3. The Power of the Spirit: How to Connect with Your Higher Self and Purpose.

It's easy to feel disoriented and overburdened in our fast-paced, frequently chaotic society. We may find ourselves yearning for a more profound sense of meaning and purpose due to the pressures of everyday life and the ceaseless stream of information and stimuli. This is when the spirit's strength, a force that is present in every one of us and just has to be recognized and used, comes into play.

Making a connection with your higher self is a life-changing experience that transcends the surface levels of reality. It explores the very center of you, revealing the strands of who you are that are frequently obscured by the outside world. Recognizing that life is made up of more than just the material and quantifiable requires an understanding of the power of the spirit. This includes the domains of consciousness, intuition, and the subtle forces that connect us to a greater purpose.

The first step in this journey is to develop self-awareness. To achieve this, you must step back from the everyday grind and inwardly focus. You can use introspective activities, mindfulness training, and meditation as doors to go deeper into your consciousness. You make room for the spirit to unfold and disclose its wisdom when you still the mind and connect with your inner self. The idea of the higher self—a transcendent part of yourself unconstrained by the confines of the material world—and the power of the spirit are intimately related. Gaining a deeper awareness of who you are requires peeling back the layers of societal conditioning and ego to connect with your higher self. Honesty, vulnerability, and a readiness to face any shadows that might be preventing you from moving forward are necessary for this process. Establishing a connection with your higher self allows you to access a wealth of wisdom and intuition. Subtle whispers, intuition, and coincidences are some of the ways the spirit speaks to you as it leads you on your journey. Since the rational mind frequently finds it difficult to understand the language of the spirit, trusting these signs is an essential part of the trip. It takes time and patience to develop the ability to follow your intuition and listen to your inner voice. Aligning with your higher self naturally leads to the discovery of your purpose. Beyond human gratification, the power of the spirit encompasses a higher sense of purpose that goes beyond personal desires. Your mission is deeply ingrained in the cosmos, and when you establish a connection with your higher self, you open up a channel for the expression of this overarching purpose.

An in-depth examination of your values, passions, and special talents is necessary to find your purpose. It's about realizing how your personal experience fits into the larger picture of existence. By enabling you to live truly and by your higher purpose, the power of the spirit cultivates a sense of fulfillment that surpasses material accomplishments. There are obstacles on the path to realizing your mission and higher self. This deep investigation may be hampered by obstacles such as ego, fear, and social expectations. The first step towards conquering these challenges is realizing they exist. Compassion, self-love, and self-reflection are effective strategies for overcoming obstacles that stand in the way of the spirit's flow within.

The path to connecting with the power of the spirit requires community and support. Being in the company of people who are on a similar path to self-discovery and purpose may be inspiring, motivating, and give you a feeling of community. Experiences and insights that are shared provide a group energy that enhances the spiritual journey's capacity for transformation.

It's critical to recognize that no single religion or spiritual tradition is exempt from the power of the spirit. Although many practices and belief systems provide useful frameworks and tools, the core of connecting with your higher self is universal. People are encouraged to investigate and understand their connection in a way that aligns with their particular experiences and beliefs due to the spirit's universal nature.

Each of us possesses the innate power of the spirit, which is just waiting to be acknowledged and welcomed. A significant journey, including self-awareness, faith in intuition, and a readiness to face and overcome internal difficulties, involves connecting with your higher self and purpose. You find a source of wisdom that directs you toward a purpose that transcends personal goals as you explore the depths of yourself. The ability to live truly, connect with your higher purpose, and make a positive impact on the world around you is all made possible by the transformative power of the spirit. Accept this trip and let the spirit's light guide you toward a life that is more purposeful and happy.

Chapter Two

The Power of Relationships: How to Attract and Nurture Positive People in Your Life

Our happiness, health, and general well-being all depend on our relationships. They provide us happiness, love, support, and company. But not every connection is advantageous and fruitful. Some may be hazardous, poisonous, and exhausting. How do we reduce or keep the negative people out of our lives while attracting and nurturing the positive ones?

Being optimistic yourself is one technique to attract positive people to you. This entails having optimism, gratitude, kindness, and civility. Positivity radiates from people in a way that makes others want to be around them. Additionally, they steer clear of rumors, judgment, and criticism, as these things turn off possible friends and partners. Having a positive outlook on life can help you draw in companions who share your goals and principles. Being sincere and real is another technique to draw in positive people. This entails staying loyal to your aims, feelings, and views about yourself. People who value their individuality and integrity are drawn to those who are genuine and honest. Additionally, they resist hiding, lying, and pretending—actions that foster mistrust and alienation. You may attract individuals who appreciate and admire you for who you are by being genuine and honest. Positivity can also be attracted by being open-minded and inquisitive. This entails having the willingness to develop, learn, and try new things. People who are adventurous, creative, and fun tend to be drawn to those who are open and curious. Additionally, they steer clear of being narrow-minded, dogmatic, and uninteresting, all of which can restrict their chances and experiences. You can meet and attract individuals who push and encourage you to broaden your horizons by being open and inquisitive. How do you maintain and grow the positive people you have drawn into your life? Being able to speak well is one strategy to foster great relationships. This calls for clarity, deference, and empathy. Understanding, resolving, and preventing disputes all depend on effective communication. Expressing your needs, wants, and expectations is also beneficial. You can cultivate healthy relationships by establishing closeness, respect, and trust through efficient communication. Offer assistance and motivation as an additional means of cultivating wholesome connections. This entails lending a hand, giving, and showing compassion. Friendship, partnership, and teamwork are built on the foundations of support and encouragement. They also support, empower, and inspire. You can cultivate healthy connections by fortifying ties, demonstrating commitment, and expressing thanks. Appreciating and celebrating one another is a third strategy for fostering happy partnerships. This entails being happy, appreciative, and complimentary. Love, friendship, and family are ignited by celebration and gratitude. They also aid in rewarding, honoring, and recognizing. You can cultivate happy, fulfilling, and loving relationships by taking the time to celebrate and express gratitude.

In summary, connections have a strong and lasting impact on our lives. They have the power to improve or worsen our health, happiness, and general well-being. As a result, it's critical to eliminate or avoid bad people in our lives and to draw in and support positive ones. People who share our values and vision can be drawn to us if we are genuine, upbeat, and honest. Effective communication, encouragement, and support, as well as celebration and appreciation, are all important components of building strong, enduring relationships.

4. The Power of Gratitude: How to Appreciate and Celebrate the Good Things in Your Life

Being grateful is the attitude of not dwelling on our shortcomings but rather being appreciative of what we do have. It's an optimistic outlook that can improve our relationships, happiness, and general well-being. Additionally, gratitude can support us in overcoming stress, hardship, and obstacles.

But how can we practice thankfulness in our day-to-day activities? The following advice can assist you in recognizing and honoring the positive aspects of your life:

- Maintain a thankfulness diary. Every day, list three things for which you are thankful. They can be little or large, like a warm day, a kind word, or an embrace. Regularly read over your journal to see how your mood has improved.

- Thank people for their contributions. Express your gratitude to strangers, coworkers, family, and friends for everything they do for you. Additionally, you can send messages, write thank-you notes, and present gifts. Expressing your gratitude to the person would lift their spirits as much as yours.
- engage in mindfulness. Be mindful of the beauty and amazement surrounding you, and stay in the present moment. You can relax your body and mind by practicing yoga, meditation, or deep breathing. Accept the thoughts, feelings, and sensations that come up without passing judgment on them.
- Cherish the good times. Don't let a nice thing pass you by too quickly. Rather, take your time and savor it thoroughly. You can also write it

down in your journal or share it with others. Your appreciation and happiness will increase if you take time to savor the good times.

- Disprove the pessimistic ideas. Avoid letting setbacks or disappointments get the better of you. Rather, look for the good or the lesson in every circumstance. You might also consider your blessings despite the adversity. You may overcome negative ideas and develop resilience by confronting them.

Being grateful is a strong and easy approach to making life better. Regular gratitude practice will help you feel more content, upbeat, and connected, as well as enable you to recognize and celebrate the positive aspects of your life.

5.The Power of Meditation: How to Calm Your Mind and Enhance Your Awareness

Although meditation has been practiced for thousands of years, it has recently become more well-known as a stress-reduction, health, and well-being tool. The practice of concentrating your attention on a certain object, feeling, or thought while letting go of distractions and judgments is known as meditation. You may improve your awareness of yourself and your environment, quiet your mind, and unwind your body with the aid of meditation.

Reducing stress and its detrimental impact on your health is one of the benefits of meditation. Numerous medical conditions, including high blood pressure, heart disease, anxiety, and depression, can be brought on by stress or made worse by it. By triggering the parasympathetic nervous system, which is in charge of the relaxation response, meditation can assist you in managing stress. This can relieve muscle tension and lower your blood pressure, respiration rate, and heart rate. Additionally, by enhancing your resilience, problem-solving abilities, and emotional control, meditation can help you deal with difficult situations.

An additional advantage of meditation is that it can improve your consciousness and awareness. The capacity to remain in the present moment without passing judgment or responding to it is known as mindfulness. You can accept things as they are and become more conscious of your thoughts, feelings, sensations, and surroundings by practicing mindfulness. Your creativity, recall, focus, and mental clarity can all be enhanced by doing this. Additionally, practicing mindfulness can lessen negative emotions like fear, anger, and sadness and help you develop positive feelings like happiness, compassion, and gratitude.

There are numerous varieties of meditation, and each has unique methods and objectives. The following are a few of the popular forms of meditation:

- Focusing your attention on a single item during meditation: such as your breath, a sound, a word, or a picture, is known as concentration meditation. This kind of meditation aims to teach your mind to focus and keep away from distractions.
- Heart-centered meditation: This kind of meditation focuses on the middle of your chest, the area that is said to be the energy center of your heart. This sort of meditation is meant to help you develop compassion, kindness, and love for both yourself and other people.
- Mindfulness meditation: entails paying attention to your thoughts,

feelings, sensations, and surroundings without passing judgment or responding in any way. This kind of meditation aims to improve your mindfulness and awareness of the here and now.

- Qigong and tai chi: are movement-based meditation techniques that incorporate breathing, concentration, and physical activity. These kinds of meditation aim to reconcile your mind and body, enhance your health, and balance your energy.

- Transcendental Meditation: This kind of meditation focuses on calming your mind and entering a profound level of relaxation by repeating a mantra, which is a word, phrase, or sound. This kind of meditation aims to help you reach a higher state of awareness and transcend your everyday consciousness.

- Walking meditation: This kind of meditation entails breathing in rhythm with your stride and focusing on your body and environment. This kind of meditation aims to help you become more in tune with nature and your body.

A quick and easy method to clear your head and become more conscious is to meditate. As long as you have a few minutes and a comfortable spot, you can meditate anytime, anywhere. To learn from an experienced teacher and gain from the energy of other meditators, you can also enroll in a class or group meditation, or use an audio or guided meditation app. You can enhance your life with greater serenity, joy, and wisdom through meditation, as well as your physical, mental, and emotional well-being.

6. The Power of Affirmations: How to Use Words to Manifest Your Desires.

Positive, present-tense words or declarations that are repeatedly repeated to support optimistic attitudes and thoughts are known as affirmations. They are a well-liked tool in positive psychology, self-help, and personal development, and they are most frequently used to improve motivation, self-assurance, and open-mindedness. Affirmations have the power to alter the narrative you tell yourself, as well as how you see the world and live. You can use affirmations as a means of drawing positive things into your life, such as a successful profession, abundant finances, or a loving relationship, by increasing your self-assurance.

A 2018 study found that repeating affirmations to oneself regularly can boost your self-esteem, help you deal with uncertainty, and increase your ability to handle stress and other challenges in life. Additionally, affirmations can help you grow and learn from setbacks, as well as draw in more possibilities. Affirmations, for instance, have been demonstrated to activate brain areas linked to enhanced self-worth. Numerous accomplished individuals have discussed the value of using positive self-talk and how it can enhance well-being and success. To boost his drive, Tony Robbins, for instance, says affirmations like "I am grateful for everything that I am and everything that I have." This comforting statement, "I'm a work in progress, and I hope that I will always be," is what Michelle Obama counts on.

How to Effectively Use Affirmations

You must adhere to a few fundamental rules to use affirmations effectively:

- Select affirmations that are consistent with your ambitions, values, and goals. Verify that they hold significance, are reasonable, and are relevant to you.
- Make use of the first person and the present tense. Say "I am" rather than "I will" or "I want," for instance. This facilitates the creation of a feeling of actuality and immediacy.
- Speak in an empowering and upbeat manner. Stay away from using derogatory terms like "not," "can't," or "don't." Say "I am confident" as an example, rather than "I am not afraid."
- Recite your affirmations out loud regularly. These can be jotted down in a journal, silently repeated in

your thoughts, spoken out, shown, or recorded, and then played again. Your subconscious mind will become more and more accustomed to them the more you repeat them.

- Your affirmations should be motivated by emotion. Just picture your feelings if your affirmations come to pass. Emotions are strong forces that influence behavior and expression.
- Incorporate other constructive activities with your affirmations. You can, for instance, journal, imagine, meditate, or take concrete steps to support your affirmations.

Affirmations for Manifestation Examples

The following are some examples of manifestation affirmations that you can use or adapt to your own needs:

- I draw my ambitions and dreams to me like a magnet.

- I'm realizing my goals.
- I reside in a fantastic home in a fantastic community.
- In my life, good things happen daily.
- Every action I take results in success.
- I am present. I am strong. I am blessed and abundant.
- I have hope for the future.
- I exude a lot of pleasant energy.
- I have the power to materialize anything I choose.
- Joy and love are my guides.
- I attract miracles like a magnet.
- My ability to manifest is strong.
- My goals in life are very clear.
- I am seeking what I am seeking.
- I cherish who I am. I sustain myself. I have confidence in myself.
- I decide to be good to myself.

- I encourage my aspirations. I support my objectives. I encourage my trip.
- I have no trouble believing in myself.
- I surround myself with uplifting individuals. I surround myself with positive people who support and motivate me to achieve my objectives.
- To accomplish my goals, I venture outside of my comfort zone.
- I'm free to put myself through challenges.

One easy and powerful technique to use words to actualize your wishes is through affirmations. As long as you have a few minutes and a cozy spot, you can practice affirmations anytime, anywhere. You can also take advantage of the collective energy of other affirmers and learn from an experienced teacher by enrolling in a class or group using an audio or guided app. You can enhance your life with more serenity, happiness, and wisdom by using affirmations to enhance your physical, mental, and emotional well-being.

Chapter Three

The Power of Visualization: How to Use Images to Create Your Reality.

By using the imagination, visualization is a mental practice that helps you achieve your goals and realize your aspirations. Using all five senses to create a vivid and realistic mental image of your desired outcome is the process of visualization. You may train your subconscious mind to focus on your objectives and take the required steps to make them a reality by doing this.

There are several advantages to visualization, including lowered stress and anxiety, increased confidence, and enhanced physical performance. You may make your objectives more accessible than ever before by using the power of your mind's eye to visualize them and build a clear path toward them.

The following actions can help you make efficient use of visualization:

- Pick a peaceful, comfortable spot where you won't be distracted or bothered by sounds as you visualize.

- Establish a goal at the outset that is precise and written in the present tense. For instance, "I am managing a profitable business" or "I am residing in my ideal home."

- Shut your eyes and unwind, both mentally and physically. To help you relax, try breathing techniques, meditation, or listening to music.

- Make your vision of yourself accomplishing your objective as realistic as you can by using all of your senses. Imagine yourself in the scene; you can even taste the flavors, smell the smells, feel the emotions, and hear the sounds.

Your visualization will be more potent the more details you include.

- To strengthen your positive picture and intention, repeat your visualization every day, especially in the morning or evening. Affirmations are encouraging words that support your objective; you can use them to improve your visualization. For instance, "I am a capable and self-assured business owner" or "I am worthy of my dream house."

- Implement strategies that support your objectives, and be receptive to opportunities and criticism. Action is necessary, and visualization catalyzes it. You can improve your motivation, creativity, and problem-solving abilities, as well as draw in the tools and people you need to reach your objective, by picturing it.

Using pictures to build your world may be done easily and effectively with visualization. As long as you have a few minutes and a cozy spot, you can practice visualization anytime, anywhere. You can also take advantage of the collective energy of other visualizers by enrolling in a class or group, using an audio or guided app, or learning from an experienced teacher. You can enhance your life with more serenity, joy, and wisdom and enhance your physical, mental, and emotional well-being by practicing visualization.

7.The Power of Action: How to Take Inspired Steps to Achieve Your Goals

The link between your aspirations and reality is action. Your aspirations will remain dreams or wishes if you do nothing. It is an action that converts your vision into real outcomes. You learn, adapt, and overcome obstacles through action. It's an action that gives you a sense of fulfillment and life.

However, not every action is equal. Certain behaviors are motivated by dread, uncertainty, or duty. Stress, annoyance, or regret could result from doing these things. Other acts are motivated by inspiration, passion, or intuition. These deeds could result in happiness, fulfillment, or achievement.

Inspired activity is the kind that is in line with your genuine passion and purpose. The kind of action that comes easily and spontaneously from your inner guidance is called inspired action. Inspired activity is the kind that fills you with enthusiasm, energy, and excitement.

How to Act with Inspiration

The following strategies will assist you in acting more inspiredly:

- Reach out to your inner compass. Inner nudges, creativity bursts, and intuitive hunches are easy to ignore. You can practice mindfulness, meditation, or journaling to make sure you don't miss anything. You can listen to your inner voice and learn how to tune it using these techniques.

- Establish SMART objectives. SMART stands for time-bound, specific, measurable, achievable, and relevant. You can track your progress, concentrate your efforts, and define your vision with the aid of SMART goals. You can also break down your lofty ambitions into smaller, more doable steps with the aid of SMART goals.

- Make a strategy of action. A document that lists the actions or steps you must take to accomplish your goal is called an action plan. You can prioritize your tasks, keep yourself on track, and organize your thoughts with the aid of an action plan. You can also find possible roadblocks and solutions with the use of an action plan.
- Do something every day. The secret to reaching your goals is consistency. Over time, even tiny daily steps can add up to a significant difference. You can also increase your momentum, self-assurance, and motivation by taking action each day. You can also overcome reluctance, fear, or procrastination by acting daily.

- Honor your accomplishments. Remember to express your gratitude and acknowledgment for your accomplishments. Celebrating your successes can encourage you to keep going, strengthen your positive behaviors, and increase your sense of self-worth. Honoring your successes might also assist you in drawing prosperity and new chances into your life.

A strong strategy for realizing your dreams and making your vision a reality is inspired action. As long as you have a clear vision, a strong intention, and an optimistic outlook, you may practice inspired action at any time or place. You can also take advantage of the collective energy of other action-takers by joining a class or group, using an audio or guided app, or learning from an experienced teacher. You can enhance your life with greater serenity, happiness, and wisdom, as well as better physical, mental, and emotional health, by taking inspired action.

8. The Power of Creativity: How to Express Your Unique Gifts and Talents

The capacity to come up with novel and inventive concepts, items, or solutions is known as creativity. Being creative is a crucial skill that can benefit you in many areas of your life, including social interaction, professional advancement, and personal improvement. You can exhibit your special talents and gifts—the innate skills or attributes that define who you are—by using your creativity. Though not everyone is aware of them, everyone possesses talents and gifts. We could have feelings of insecurity, uncertainty, or fear when we want to showcase our abilities to others. Sometimes, we might not even be conscious of our abilities or inventive ways to apply our gifts.

Thankfully, there are methods available to assist you in expressing your abilities and letting your creativity run wild. The following advice will help you get started:

- Investigate your passions and interests. Following your passion and curiosity is one of the finest ways to discover your gifts and abilities. What activities, knowledge, or experiences do you enjoy? What gives you a sense of fulfillment, happiness, or life? These are the hints that can help you discover your abilities and skills. See what inspires your creativity by experimenting with various interests, pastimes, or themes.

- Ask for advice and motivation. Getting input and inspiration from others is another way to identify and utilize your skills. You can get advice and ideas about your areas of strength and growth from friends, family, coaches, mentors, and teachers. To gain knowledge from their experiences and accomplishments, you might also search for mentors, role models, or examples of people who possess comparable abilities and gifts to yourself. Books, articles, podcasts, videos, and other informational resources that can assist you in enhancing your skills and abilities can also serve as inspiration.
- Try new things and push yourself. Taking on new challenges and experimenting with your skills is a third approach to letting your creativity run wild and showcasing

your abilities. You can challenge yourself, try new things, take chances, create objectives, and become involved in initiatives or competitions that will push your limits. You can also try expressing your skills and abilities in other ways, using different instruments or forms, including writing, speaking, painting, dancing, singing, coding, or inventing. You may explore and express your creativity to a greater extent the more you experiment and push yourself.

- Give credit to your work and share it with others. Sharing your work and appreciating your effort is a fourth technique to showcase your abilities. You can receive comments, encouragement, or acknowledgment by sharing your work with others—friends, family, classmates, or online groups, for example. You can also make a difference or have a good impact by sharing your work with the public through publishing, performing, exhibiting, or selling it. By recognizing, valuing, and celebrating your abilities and gifts and how they can help you and others, you can also add value to your contribution.

Using your creativity to express your special abilities and gifts is a powerful technique. If you have a clear goal, a strong aim, and an optimistic outlook, you can be creative anywhere and at any time. You can also make use of the collective energy of other creative individuals by enrolling in a class or group, using an audio or guided app, or learning from an experienced teacher. Your life can be made more peaceful, joyful, and wise by being more creative, which can also help you maintain better physical, mental, and emotional health.

9.The Power of Joy: How to Find and Do What Makes You Happy.

Joy is an internalized state of profound delight and well-being. Joy is an internal state of mind that is independent of external conditions. Choosing joy is something you can do every day, no matter what is going on in your life. Another ability that you may develop and get better at is joy.

What brings you joy, and how can you pursue it? Many people's goals are centered around this question. Several circumstances can influence happiness. People commonly define it as encompassing happy emotions and life satisfaction. Your relationships, values, personality, health, interests, and purpose are a few of these variables.

While everyone finds joy and happiness in various ways, certain universal patterns might guide you in identifying and pursuing your sources of happiness. The following advice can assist you in identifying and pursuing your happiness:

- Determine your passions and areas of strength. Using your talents and passions to make a significant contribution to something worthwhile is one of the finest ways to discover joy and happiness. What are the things you enjoy doing, find fulfilling, or find important? In what ways can you apply them to improve your life and the lives of others? You might feel more joy and fulfillment when your abilities and passions are in line with your mission.

- Give thanks and acknowledgement. Having thankfulness and appreciation for what you have and what you experience is another way to be happy. Recognizing and appreciating the positive aspects of your life, no matter how great or tiny, material or immaterial, is the act of being grateful. The act of showing gratitude to others or oneself is called appreciation. By showing appreciation and thankfulness to others, you can improve your relationships, develop a positive outlook, and bring more joy and abundance into your life.

- Foster happy feelings and connections. Cultivating happy feelings and relationships is a third strategy for finding joy and happiness. Positive emotions, such as joy, love, peace, and enthusiasm, are those that make you feel good Positive partnerships are the connections that give you a sense of understanding, worth, and support. You may improve your resilience, elevate your mood, and fill your life with more joy and happiness by fostering good emotions and relationships.

- Take part in the things that make you happy. Taking part in joyful and fulfilling activities is a fourth strategy to achieve joy and happiness. Whether they are pastimes, sports, the arts, or leisure, these are the things that give you a sense of life, happiness, and fulfillment. You can challenge yourself, have fun, and express your creativity by doing things that make you happy.
- Spread your happiness and joy to others. Sharing your happiness and

joy with others is a fifth approach to finding it. Giving, lending a hand, or celebrating with others are some ways to achieve this. You can double your joy and happiness and spread positivity and bonds by sharing your joy and happiness with others.

Discovering pleasure and joy is a lifelong journey that starts with a set of actions that will eventually bring you there. But remember that happiness and joy can mean various things to different people. Examine how your life is going right now, gauge how happy you are, and decide on a course of action that will probably make you happier.

Chapter Four

The Power of Love: How to Give and Receive Unconditional Love.

One of the strongest and most intense feelings that people may have is love. Love has the power to heal our wounds, ease our sorrows, spur us on to new heights, and fill our lives with joy, happiness, and fulfillment. In addition, as we negotiate the highs and lows of relationships, expectations, and disagreements, love may be difficult, complicated, and even painful at times. Unconditional love is among the best and most desired types of love. Love that is given and accepted without any restrictions, judgments, or expectations is known as unconditional love. It is the kind of love that, rather than attempting to control or alter the other person, welcomes and accepts them for who they are. It is the kind of love that gives freely and forgives without expecting anything in return.

The love that exists between parents and children or between pets and their owners is sometimes linked to unconditional love. Unconditional love, however, can also exist in friendships, romantic partnerships, and other kinds of relationships. In addition to enhancing our mental, emotional, and physical well-being, unconditional love may fill our lives with greater joy, tranquility, and wisdom.

How can we love each other without conditions? Many people want to know the answer to this question because they want to encounter this kind of love at some point in their lives. Even if it might not be straightforward, unconditional love is achievable with effort and direction. The following advice can assist

you in showing and receiving
unconditional love:

- Let everyone be themselves and be
  yourself. Being true to yourself and
  others is essential to receiving
  unconditional love. Don't try to
  pass for someone you're not, and
  don't keep your actual desires,
  feelings, or thoughts to yourself.
  Never expect someone else to meet
  your requirements, be flawless, or
  live up to your expectations. Honor
  and value your individuality as well
  as the diversity of others, and
  rejoice in the distinctions that
  define who you are.
- Be kind and respectful when you
  speak. Respectful and kind
  communication is another essential
  component of unconditional love.
  Communicate your needs, wants,
  and opinions in a direct,
  considerate, and helpful manner.

Listen to people with openness, curiosity, and empathy. Refrain from judging, accusing, or condemning other people, as well as from assuming anything about them. Instead of trying to convince or change others, try to understand and embrace them.

- Donate without anticipating anything in return. Giving without expecting is the third element of unconditional love. Give others your time, care, support, attention, or assistance without anticipating anything in return. Donate not out of obligation or expectation of reciprocation, but because you feel compelled to. Don't compare, compete, or keep score with other people. Don't give with any conditions, demands, or hidden agendas. Give liberally and freely, and relish the giving process itself.

- Let go and extend forgiveness. Forgiveness and letting go are the four essentials of unconditional love. Accept forgiveness for the errors, injuries, and disappointments you and other people may have experienced in the past. Let go of any anger, bitterness, or resentment that might be preventing you from completely and freely loving. Don't be resentful, seek retribution, or focus on the bad. Don't let the past define you or your relationships; instead, use it as a lesson. Focus on the here and now, and move on with dignity and kindness.
- Exercise appreciation and thankfulness. Developing appreciation and thankfulness is the fifth essential of unconditional love. No matter how big or tiny, material or intangible, the love you

have and receive in your life should make you feel thankful. Respect those who show you love and affection, be they friends, family, lovers, or strangers. Give thanks and appreciation to yourself and other people on a regular or sporadic basis, either orally or nonverbally. Don't take for granted the positive things in your life; instead, recognize and appreciate them.

Unconditional love is a journey that takes time, courage, and compassion to give and receive. Even if it's not always simple, it's always worthwhile. You may grow more unconditional love in your life and spread it to others by implementing the advice in this article. You can enhance your life with greater serenity, joy, and wisdom, as well as better physical, mental, and emotional health, by showing unconditional love to yourself.

10. The Power of Compassion: How to Care for Yourself and Others.

When we see someone else suffer, we experience compassion, which is the warmth and empathy that make us want to take away their suffering. Both those who give and those who receive compassion benefit from compassion. Our relationships, general well-being, and mental, emotional, and physical health can all be enhanced by compassion.

We can be compassionate toward one another or ourselves. The capacity for self-compassion is the capacity to show ourselves the same consideration and understanding that we would show a friend who is going through a difficult moment. Self-compassion can boost our resilience, happiness, and self-esteem while assisting us in managing stress, failure, or criticism. The capacity to acknowledge and react to another person's suffering without passing judgment or assigning blame is known as compassion. Having compassion for others can improve our relationships with them, promote cooperation and trust, and lessen conflict and violence.

How do we develop and put compassion into practice? Many people want to know the answer to this issue to lead more meaningful and compassionate lives. Some people may naturally possess compassion, but others may need to develop and exercise it. Fortunately, with the right direction and instruction, compassion is a talent that can be improved. The following advice will assist you in developing and using compassion:

- Engage in mindfulness. Being mindful means being aware of what is happening at the moment without letting ideas, feelings, or sensations divert you. By assisting us in paying attention to our own and others' needs and feelings without passing judgment or responding in kind, mindfulness can help us develop compassion. Additionally, practicing mindfulness can lessen stress, improve empathy, and help us control our emotions. By breathing, practicing mindfulness, or engaging in any activity that demands your complete focus and awareness, you can cultivate this mentality.
- Embrace kindness with compassion. The emotion of warmth, friendliness, and goodwill toward oneself and others is known as loving-kindness. By encouraging

the generation of pleasant feelings and thoughts and the overcoming of negative ones, loving kindness can assist us in developing compassion. We may improve our relationships, mend our wounds, and forgive ourselves and others with the use of loving-kindness. Repetition of affirmations or words such as "May I be happy, healthy, and peaceful" or "May you be free from suffering, pain, and fear" will help you cultivate loving-kindness.

- Exercise appreciation and thankfulness. The emotions of appreciation and thankfulness for the positive things in our lives, no matter how great or tiny, material or immaterial, are known as gratitude and appreciation. By assisting us in recognizing and appreciating the goodness and generosity of others as well as ourselves, as well as the beauty and abundance of the world, gratitude and appreciation can foster compassion in us. We can also feel happier, more satisfied, and more optimistic when we express our gratitude and appreciation. You can cultivate appreciation and thankfulness by keeping a journal, saying "thank you," or lending a helpful hand to others.

- Exercise selflessness and service. The deeds of assisting, providing, or enhancing the welfare of others without anticipating anything in return are acts of altruism and service. By enabling us to act on our goals and compassionate thoughts and change the world for the better, altruism and service can aid in the cultivation of compassion. Serving others and being altruistic can also help us reach our full potential and feel more purposeful and meaningful. Altruism and service can be demonstrated through volunteering, giving, or endorsing a cause that you find meaningful.

- Practice perspective-taking and empathy. The capacity to comprehend and share the emotions, ideas, and experiences of others as well as to adopt their perspective is known as empathy and perspective-taking. By enabling us to relate to, connect with, and recognize the diversity and complexity of others, empathy and perspective-taking can support the development of compassion in us. In addition to lowering our biases, prejudices, and stereotypes, empathy and perspective-taking can also help us become more accepting and tolerant of others. By asking questions, listening to people, or visualizing how they feel, think, or see things, you can work on your empathy and perspective-taking skills. Compassion cultivation and practice are continuous processes that include intention, focus, and action. Even though it's not always simple, the rewards are constant. You can improve your compassion for both yourself and other people, as well as add more wisdom, joy, and peace to your life, by implementing these suggestions.

11. The Power of Forgiveness: How to Heal and Let Go of the Past.

Letting go of our grudges, ill will, or hatred toward someone who has wronged us in the past is an act of forgiveness. To be forgiven is to release oneself from the negative feelings that bind us to the past, not to forget or justify the hurt that was done to us. We can choose to forgive to mend our hearts and go on with our lives.

Why is it crucial to forgive?

Our emotional, mental, and physical health all depend on our ability to forgive. Research has indicated that harboring hatred and grudges might raise our blood pressure, stress levels, and risk of heart disease. Additionally, it may harm our immune system, sleep patterns, and mental abilities. However, forgiving is a skill that can help us feel less stressed and have lower blood pressure and pulse rates. Additionally, it can enhance our ability to think, sleep quality, and immune system.

Our relationships and happiness both depend on forgiveness. It can be detrimental to our relationships, communication, and trust with others to harbor grudges and resentment. Additionally, it may increase our susceptibility to worry, despair, and rage. However, forgiving others can improve our connection, communication, and sense of trust. Additionally, it can increase our joy, optimism, and compassion.

How can we put forgiveness into practice?

Becoming forgiving is a process that could take patience and work. While it is feasible and satisfying, it is not necessarily straightforward. The following actions can assist us in cultivating forgiveness:

- Recognize the pain. Recognizing the harm that was done to us and how it affected us is the first step. Regarding what transpired and how it affected us, we must be truthful and grounded in reality. We must not repress or reject the hurt, rage, or despair we experience; instead, we must allow ourselves to feel them.

- Recognize the other individual. Understanding the other person who harmed us and their viewpoint is the second stage. We must make an effort to understand them and take into account their circumstances, goals, and motivations. We must never forget that they are fallible human beings with their shortcomings. We must acknowledge that their actions might not have been motivated by

evil or malice, but rather by
ignorance, fear, or grief.
- Decide to pardon. Choosing to
  forgive the other person and let go
  of your resentment, wrath, or
  bitterness is the third step. To let go
  of the bad feelings and embrace the
  good ones, we must consciously
  and unconsciously choose to do so.
  We must never forget that
  forgiveness is a sign of courage and
  strength rather than weakness. We
  must never forget that forgiveness
  is for us, not for the other person.
- Please accept my forgiveness.
  Giving the other person your
  forgiveness—either orally or
  nonverbally—is the fourth step. We
  must express to one another our
  choice to forgive and our readiness
  to go forward. Without anticipating
  anything in return, we must be
  genuine and courteous. It's

important to understand that
offering forgiveness does not
always entail making amends or
mending the relationship; rather, it
just means ending one chapter and
beginning a new one.

- Ask for pardon. Asking for
  forgiveness—verbally or
  nonverbally—from others or
  ourselves is the fifth step. We must
  own up to our mistakes and accept
  the potential harm they may have
  caused to others or ourselves. In
  addition to expressing our regret
  and guilt, we must seek
  forgiveness. We must be truthful
  and modest, without pointing
  fingers or offering justifications.
  We must understand that asking for
  forgiveness does not guarantee that
  we will be granted it; rather, it
  simply indicates that we are
  prepared to grow and change.

One of the most effective ways to move beyond and heal is through forgiveness. As long as you have a clear aim, an optimistic outlook, and a caring heart, you can practice forgiveness anywhere and at any time. You can also take advantage of the collective energy of other forgivers by enrolling in a class or group, using an audio or guided program, or learning from an experienced teacher. You can enhance your life with greater serenity, joy, and wisdom, as well as better physical, mental, and emotional health, by practicing forgiveness.

12. The Power of Resilience: How to Overcome Challenges and Adversity.

Adversity and hardships abound in life, putting our resolve and fortitude to the test. Whatever the challenge—a personal crisis, a career setback, or a pandemic—we are all susceptible to setbacks that can deflate our confidence and interfere with our plans. How can we triumph over these difficulties and misfortunes and come out stronger and smarter? Resilience holds the key to the solution. The capacity to overcome adversity and adjust to change is called resilience. It is about flourishing in the face of misfortune, not just getting by. It is possible to learn and get better at resilience through practice. We can overcome challenges, manage stress, and accomplish our objectives with resilience.

How may resilience be practiced and developed? The following techniques can assist us in strengthening and increasing our resilience:

- Maintain an optimistic outlook. Resilience is built on a positive outlook. It entails having a growth attitude, a purpose, and an optimistic outlook. Having an optimistic outlook can assist us in finding purpose in our work, viewing obstacles as opportunities, and learning from our mistakes. We can practice mindfulness, affirmations, and gratitude to develop a positive mindset.

- Cultivate solid connections. Resilience is supported by strong relationships. They entail surrounding yourself with supportive, understanding, and caring individuals. We can feel less alone, more respected, and more motivated when we have strong relationships. Strong relationships require empathetic communication, competent problem-solving, and the willingness to ask for assistance when needed.

- Attend to your own needs. Resilience is fueled by self-care. It entails looking after our mental, emotional, and physical well-being. Self-care enables us to feel happier, have more energy, and experience less stress. We may take care of ourselves by exercising frequently, eating sensibly, getting enough sleep, and unwinding.
- Accept challenges. Resilience is sparked by challenges. They entail overcoming obstacles, taking chances, and moving outside our comfort zones. We can learn, develop, and get better through challenges. We may overcome

> obstacles by being proactive, making plans, and setting reasonable objectives.

- Adapt to hardship. The best teacher of resilience is adversity. It entails going through adversity, suffering, or loss. We can develop perspective, wisdom, and strength through adversity. We can think back on what transpired, what we discovered, and what we could have done differently to learn from hardship.

One effective strategy for overcoming obstacles and misfortune is resilience. As long as you have a positive outlook, a clear vision, and a strong intention, you may exercise resilience anywhere and at any time. You can also take advantage of the collective energy of other resilient individuals by enrolling in a class or group, using an audio or guided app, or learning from an experienced teacher.

Your life can be enhanced, and your physical, mental, and emotional well-being can be enhanced with resilience.

Chapter Five

The Power of Growth: How to Learn and Evolve from Your Experiences.

The process of evolving, bettering, and building oneself and one's life is called growth. Progress is necessary for our well-being, prosperity, and contentment. As we encounter a variety of opportunities, difficulties, and experiences throughout our lives, growth is also unavoidable. How can we use our experiences as catalysts for growth, allowing us to grow and learn from them? The following advice will help you maximize your growth potential:

- Embrace a growing mentality. The idea that you can improve your skills and potential via work, feedback, and education is known as a growth mindset. You may seek out new possibilities, accept difficulties, and learn from mistakes if you have a growth mentality. You can also get rid of fixed or restricting thoughts like "I can't do this" or "I'm not good enough" by adopting a growth mindset. Setting difficult yet reasonable objectives, practicing positive self-talk, and acknowledging and celebrating your accomplishments are all ways to cultivate a development mindset.

- Think back on your past encounters. Thinking carefully and analytically about your experiences and the lessons you might draw from them is the act of reflection. You can develop wisdom, perspective, and understanding through reflection. You can discover your areas of strength, weakness, and growth by reflecting on yourself. Write in a journal, pose questions to yourself, or get input from others as ways to reflect on your experiences. Apply what you've learned.

- Applying what you've learned to enhance your performance, abilities, or results is known as application. The application can assist you in measuring your progress, verifying your comprehension, and consolidating your information. Applying yourself can also help you find solutions to issues, create value, and explore new opportunities. You can use what you've learned by taking on challenging projects or activities, trying new things, and experimenting with different approaches.
- Seek new experiences. Because they expose you to novel knowledge, concepts, or viewpoints, fresh experiences are the wellspring of personal

development. You can broaden your horizons, talents, and expertise by gaining new experiences. You can also increase your motivation, inventiveness, and curiosity by gaining new experiences. You can travel, meet new people, read, watch, or listen to something new to seek out new experiences.

- Accept change. Growth leads to change since it signifies that you have transitioned from one state to another. Depending on how you view and handle change, it can have either a positive or negative effect. You can adapt, develop, and transform with the aid of change. You can get over complacency, dullness, and stagnation by embracing change. You can be adaptable, positive, and open-minded to welcome change.

One of the most effective ways to grow from your experiences is to learn and adapt. As long as you have a clear objective, a positive attitude, and a clear vision, you may practice growth anywhere, at any time. You can also make use of the collective energy of other learners by enrolling in a class or group, using an audio or guided app, or learning from an experienced teacher. You can enhance your life and improve your physical, mental, and emotional well-being by growing.

13. The Power of Balance: How to Harmonize Your Energy Centers and Aspects of Life.

The state of harmony and balance between various energies, elements, or facets of existence is known as balance. Achieving balance can lead to the best possible health, happiness, and well-being. Additionally, balance can support us in overcoming obstacles, stress, and change.

Achieving harmony in our energy centers and life elements is one method to attain balance. The locations in our bodies where energy flows and collects are known as energy centers. Another name for them is chakras, from the Sanskrit word meaning "wheels." Our body is composed of seven primary chakras, each of which represents a distinct facet of our mental, emotional, physical, and spiritual well-being. The domains or sectors that comprise our lives—work, family, friends, interests, etc.—are known as aspects of life.

We experience vitality, alignment, and fulfillment when our energy centers and other facets of life are in harmony. When they are out of balance, we could experience fatigue, confusion, and discontent. Thus, it's critical to keep a healthy balance between our energy centers and other facets of our lives to harmonize them.

The following advice can assist you in balancing your energy centers and other facets of your life:

Determine your life's energy centers and facets. Finding your energy centers and life's elements, along with their interrelationships, is the first step. The table below can be used as a guide:

Table

Where is the Energy Center? The health aspect of color Aspects of Life Root Chakra Spine Base: Red Stability,

Survivability, and Physical Security money, house, and job

Chakra Sacral Orange below the navel Expression of emotions, inventiveness, and enjoyment Hobbies, sexuality, and relationships

Sun Chakra Plexus Yellow above the navel: willpower, self-assurance, objectives, successes, and self-worth

Heart Chakra, Chest Chakra, and Green Love, kindness, and understanding to friends, family, and the community

The blue base of the throat, or the throat chakra Verification, expression, and communication Speech, viewpoints, and convictions

Chakra of the Third Eye In between the eyebrows Indigovision, insight, and intuition Dreams, creativity, and discernment

Violet Crown Chakra at the top of the head: transcendence, spirituality, and connectedness Meaning, purpose, and faith

Evaluate your life's facets and energy centers. Assessing the balance or imbalance of your energy centers and life's facets is the second phase. The **following queries can serve as a guide for you:**

Questions about Energy Centers

Base Chakra In what ways does your life feel solid, safe, and secure? Are your basic requirements being met by the resources you have? Do you find your job, house, and career fulfilling?

Chakra Sacral Are you able to freely and healthily express your emotions? Do you encourage your passion and creativity? Do you feel happy and content in your life?

Sun Chakra Plexus Do you feel powerful and confident in yourself? Do you work toward your ambitions and goals? Do you feel good about yourself and confident?

Chakra of the Heart Do you truly love everyone, even yourself? Do you treat yourself and other people with empathy and compassion? Do you have ties that are fulfilling and encouraging in your life?

Grasping Chakra Do you speak with honesty and clarity? Do you express yourself and tell the truth? Do you listen to and respect other people?

Chakra of the Third Eye Do you heed your inner guidance and have faith in your intuition? Do you know exactly where you want your life to go? Do you try to find and acquire fresh information and wisdom?

The Crown Chakra Do you sense a connection to a source or greater power? Do you feel that your life has significance and purpose? Do you lead a spiritual or religious life?

Stabilize your energy centers and life's elements. The third phase involves harmonizing and balancing your life's aspects and energy centers. The following techniques can serve as a reference:

Table

Method Overview: Meditation Focusing on a certain object, feeling, or thought while letting go of distractions and judgments is the practice of meditation. By activating, cleansing, and balancing your energy centers, meditation can assist you in achieving balance. You can focus your meditation on one energy center at a time or on all of them. Additionally, you can employ particular sounds, mantras, or affirmations that are associated with each energy center, such as "I am love" for the heart chakra or "I am safe" for the root chakra.

Yoga is a physical and mental discipline that combines breathing techniques and postures. Your energy centers can be stimulated, opened, and balanced with the help of yoga. Yoga poses that focus on each energy center separately or all at once can be practiced. To control and balance your energy flow, you can also employ certain breathing exercises like ujjayi breath or alternate nostril breathing.

Crystal Therapy Using naturally occurring crystals or stones with particular qualities, frequencies, or hues is known as crystal healing. By amplifying, clearing, and balancing your energy centers, crystal healing can assist you in achieving balance. For example, amethyst is appropriate for the crown chakra and red jasper for the root chakra. You can also use stones that correspond to the color or quality of each energy center. The crystals can be worn as jewelry or accessories, or placed on or close to the appropriate energy center. Using aromatherapy Using natural oils or essences with particular fragrances, effects, or advantages is known as aromatherapy. Your energy centers can be calmed, stimulated, or balanced with the use of aromatherapy. For example, frankincense is good for the crown chakra, and lavender is good for the throat chakra. You can utilize oils or essences that correspond with the energy center's purpose or mood. You can apply the scents to your skin or clothing, inhale them, or distribute them in the air. Utilizing Colors in Therapy Using colors with particular meanings, impacts, or associations is known as color therapy. Your energy centers can be enhanced, harmonized, or balanced with the aid of color therapy. You can choose colors that represent each chakra's energy center, for example, indigo for the third eye chakra and red for the root chakra. You can wear the colors, surround yourself with them, or picture them.

Retain your equilibrium. Maintaining your equilibrium and keeping all facets of your life and your energy centers in harmony is the fourth phase. To do this, use the table.

Method Overview

Keep an eye on your life and energies. Keep a watch on your emotions, moods, and energy levels, and take note of any shifts or variations. Observe the circumstances, events, and results in your life and take note of any patterns or trends. Keep an eye out for any imbalanced signs or symptoms, such as exhaustion, stress, or disease, as well as any growth possibilities or obstacles, including new experiences, objectives, or interpersonal relationships.

Modify your life and energy. Restore your harmony and balance by making any required adjustments to your energy centers and other facets of your life. To balance your energy centers, use any of the aforementioned techniques or any other that seems right for you. To balance your elements of life, make use of any tools or techniques that work for you, such as delegation, planning, and prioritizing. Pay attention to your energies and life's necessities, and be proactive, adaptive, and flexible.

Savor your vitality and existence. Enjoy the harmony and balance that come from appreciating and celebrating your energy centers and other facets of life. Thank you and be grateful for your life and energy and how they sustain and enhance you. Share your compassion and love for others, as well as for how they inspire and connect with you. Express gratitude and delight for your vitality and life and how they enable and satisfy you. Achieving optimal health, well-being, and happiness may be gratifying and meaningful when your energy centers and life's facets are balanced. As long as you have a clear aim, an optimistic outlook, and a caring heart, you can practice balancing anytime and anywhere. You can also take advantage of the collective energy of other balancers by joining a class or group, using an audio or guided app, or learning from an experienced teacher. You can enhance your life with greater serenity, joy, and wisdom and enhance your physical, mental, and emotional well-being by achieving balance.

14. The Power of Nature: How to Use Renewable Energy Sources to Protect the Planet.

Climate change, the phenomenon of rising global temperatures and extreme weather events brought on by the buildup of greenhouse gases in the atmosphere, is one of the most pressing and significant issues facing humanity today. Burning fossil fuels like coal, oil, and gas to create energy for industry, transportation, and other uses is the primary source of these greenhouse gases. In addition to being bad for the environment, fossil fuels are limited and unsustainable since they will eventually run out.

Fortunately, renewable energy sources offer a solution to this issue. Natural resources such as the sun, wind, water, biomass, and geothermal heat are numerous and constantly renewed, and they are the source of renewable energy sources. Renewable energy sources are safer and cleaner for the environment than fossil fuels since they produce little or no greenhouse emissions or other pollutants. Renewable energy sources can have economic and social benefits, as they can create jobs, lower energy costs, enhance energy access, and improve energy security.

How can we save the environment by using renewable energy sources? The following actions can hasten the shift to a future powered by renewable energy:

- Boost the proportion of renewable energy sources in the world's energy mix. The United Nations estimates that now 29% of the world's electricity is generated by renewable energy sources; however, to mitigate the worst effects of climate change, this percentage must rise to at least 90% by 2050. To do this, we must increase our investments in renewable energy technologies and boost their capacity, efficiency, and dependability. Examples of these technologies include solar panels, wind turbines, hydroelectric dams, biomass facilities, and geothermal systems. In addition, we must gradually phase out subsidies for fossil fuels and enact laws and policies that encourage the advancement and use of renewable energy sources.

- Boost the distribution and integration of renewable energy sources. The variable and intermittent nature of renewable energy is a barrier since it is dependent on the intensity and availability of natural resources like wind and sunlight, which can fluctuate across time and space. Demand response, energy storage, and smart grids must all be used to better integrate and distribute renewable energy to meet this challenge. Smart grids are networks that balance the supply and demand of energy by using digital technology to monitor and control the flow of electricity from various sources and places. The technique of holding extra energy and releasing it when needed is known as energy storage. Examples of this type of storage include hydrogen, batteries, and pumped hydro. The process of modifying energy output or consumption—for example, by employing smart meters, appliances, or other gadgets—to correspond with the cost or availability of energy is known as demand response.

- Encourage the use of renewable energy. Promoting the adoption and use of renewable energy through increased participation, awareness, and education is another action we can take to employ renewable energy sources to safeguard the environment. Through the media, campaigns, or events, we can increase public awareness of the costs and hazards associated with fossil fuels as well as the advantages and benefits of renewable energy. By utilizing materials, classes, or programs, we may educate ourselves and others about the science and technology of renewable energy, as well as the opportunities and talents it offers. We can support renewable energy projects, initiatives, or organizations, or we can use renewable energy products, services, or solutions to contribute to the renewable energy movement.

Not only is it necessary to use renewable energy sources to safeguard the environment, but it is also a chance. We can make the environment greener, cleaner, and more sustainable for present and future generations by utilizing the power of nature.

15. The Power of Good Energy: How to Live a More Positive, Healthy and Fulfilling Life.

The vitality, excitement, and optimism that result from leading a happy, healthy, and purposeful life are known as good energy. We can overcome obstacles, accomplish our goals, and savor every moment while in good energy. Positive, abundant, and happy energy can also draw more of it into our lives.

How can we lead happier, healthier, and more satisfying lives? The following advice can assist you in utilizing positive energy:

- Consider the bright side. The practice of expecting the best and seeing the positive side of circumstances is known as positive thinking. We can lengthen our lives, strengthen our immune systems, and reduce stress by practicing positive thinking. We can enhance our relationships, professions, and happiness by adopting a positive mindset. We can engage in mindfulness, affirmations, and gratitude practices to think positively.

- Consume wholesome food. The practice of selecting foods that are good for our body, mind, and soul is known as healthy eating. Eating healthily can improve our happiness, help us avoid disease, and help us maintain our weight. Eating well can also make us feel fuller, more attentive, and more invigorated. We can eat a balanced diet, stay away from processed foods, and drink lots of water to stay healthy.
- Engage in regular exercise. The practice of exercising our bodies in ways that enhance our mental, emotional, and physical well-being

is known as regular exercise. Frequent exercise can enhance blood circulation, metabolism, digestion, and the strength of our muscles, bones, and organs. Frequent exercise also facilitates the release of endorphins, which are happy-making natural substances. To exercise frequently, we should choose an activity we enjoy doing, like dance, yoga, walking, or jogging, and commit to doing it for at least 30 minutes three times a week.

- Rest well at night. Sleeping well means making it a habit to receive the recommended amount and quality of sleep each night. We can heal our cells, regain our vitality, and solidify our memories with the aid of a healthy sleep schedule. Good sleep can also help us regulate our hormones, emotions, and appetite. We can maintain a regular sleep schedule, abstain from alcohol, caffeine, and devices just before bed, and make sure our sleeping space is cozy and dark.

- Learn new stuff. The habit of broadening our knowledge, abilities, and interests is learning new things. Acquiring new knowledge can help us become more confident, creative, and mentally active. Acquiring knowledge can also assist us in finding fresh opportunities, resolving issues, and adding value. We can enroll in a course, read, watch, or listen to anything new, or we can join a hobby organization to learn new things.
- Enjoy yourself. Having fun is the practice of doing things that make us happy, pleasurable, and giggle. Having fun can facilitate social

interaction, relaxation, and recharging. Additionally, having fun can help us communicate our individuality, passions, and goals. We can play games, watch movies, or listen to music, or we can do something different like volunteer, travel, or pick up a new language to have fun.

- Show kindness. Being kind is the habit of treating oneself and others with respect, compassion, and generosity. Our well-being, pleasure, and sense of self-worth can all be enhanced by kindness. Additionally, kindness can foster mutual respect, cooperation, and peace. To be kind, we can take care of ourselves, show empathy and forgiveness, and do good deeds for others or ourselves, like offering a gift, an embrace, or a compliment.

Achieving a more contented, healthy, and pleasant existence is a worthwhile endeavor that will help both ourselves and other people. As long as you have a clear objective, an upbeat mindset, and positive energy, you may practice these habits anywhere and at any time. To learn from an experienced teacher and gain from the collective energy of other good, healthy, and fulfilling people, you can also join a class or group or utilize a guided app or podcast. Enhancing your physical, mental, and emotional well-being and adding value to your life can be achieved by leading a happier, healthier, and more satisfying existence.

Conclusion

Though this book has come to a conclusion, your journey is far from over. You now know the value of positive energy and how to lead a happier, healthier, and more satisfying existence. Additionally, you now know about the several routines, exercises, and approaches that can support you in developing positive energy and using it to enhance your life and yourself. However, education is insufficient. You must put what you've learned into practice and incorporate it into your everyday activities. Your positive energy must continue to flow; you must not allow it to wane or stagnate. You must never stop learning, developing, and growing; you must never accept anything less than what you are due.

How are you able to accomplish that? Here are some pointers to help you maintain your positive vibes:
Examine your development and accomplishments. Spend some time thinking back on your progress and personal development. Be proud of yourself, and acknowledge and appreciate your accomplishments. Acknowledge and value the positive energy you have drawn to yourself and others, as well as the benefits it has brought.
Establish fresh objectives and difficulties. Aim for where you want to be instead of stopping at where you are. Establish new objectives and tasks that are in line with your passion and purpose and that will inspire and encourage you. Push yourself beyond your comfort zone and investigate uncharted territory. Don't allow your positive energy to stagnate. Keep it flowing.

Ask for advice and assistance. Instead of isolating yourself, make connections with people who share your beliefs and objectives. Consult your friends, relatives, mentors, or coaches for advice and encouragement. You can also gain knowledge from their experiences and perspectives. Be in the company of upbeat, encouraging people who can guide you toward your objectives and help you develop. Don't let your positive energy fade; instead, spread it to others. Continue to grow and learn. Avoid complacency by remaining modest and inquisitive. Continue to learn and develop your interests, abilities, and knowledge. Take a course, sign up for a hobby organization, or read, watch, or listen to anything new. Seek out and acquire fresh information and insight to help you strengthen your positive energy. Keep an open mind to new ideas and developments, and keep your positive vibes current.

Enjoy life and have pleasure. Instead of being anxious, try to be content and at ease. Enjoy life, have fun, and pursue your happiness. Engage in gaming, film viewing, or music listening. Take a trip, lend a hand, and pick up a language. Communicate your ideas, feelings, and goals. Revel in the delight and joy that your positive energy gives, and hold onto it.

You possess the ability to design and lead a happier, healthier, and more satisfying life. You are capable of creating and sustaining positive energy, which you may then channel to better your life and yourself. You have the ability to change the world for the better and motivate others to follow in your footsteps.

You possess positive energy. Make good and sensible use of it.